Dedicated to the parents who never gave

up on their dream to fill their homes with

the life, love, and laughter of children.

And to the children for whom this book

was written:

May you have a joyful and interesting life,

and remember ...

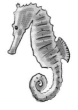

You are wonderfully made!

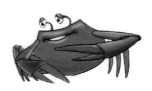

ISBN-13: 978-0-692-24536-1

Text copyright © 2014 by Carien Myburgh

Illustrations by MikeMotz.com

Illustrations copyright © 2014 by ObO Books Inc.

Published 2015 by ObO Books Inc.

Distributed via amazon.com

Foreword

Issues of disclosure to a child conceived with donor egg and sperm are often difficult to deal with. The question arises about whether to tell the child about their origins and if so, how?

This book explains this issue in simple terms, easy for a child to understand. It can be used as a tool to initiate the conversation about the child's origins and help them develop comfort with their identity.

Rinku Mehta, MD, FACOG
Board Certified in Reproductive Endocrinology and Infertility

'The Dancing Fish and the Clever Crab' provides a wonderful platform to open the discussion of how a donor can help a couple reach their dreams of having a family. As an experienced infertility counselor with a thorough understanding of the psychological needs of children, Carien (Reen) Myburgh, LPC has written this book in a manner that is easy for young ones to understand and connect with. This book captures the core meaning of what makes us parents and how "non-traditional" families are created.

Having worked in the infertility field for over 18 years, I know this book will serve as a valuable resource to many parents!

Jan Mazraani, RDMS
Donor Coordinator

This book belongs to:

We are so happy to have you

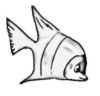

in our life!

From: _____

Date: _____

The Dancing Fish
and the
Clever Crab

In a part of the ocean where the waters are warm, and sunlight flows lazily all the way to the starfish and plants, live many kinds of beautiful and interesting sea creatures.

Among these beautiful creatures are the Dancing Fish. They are called Dancing Fish because little offspring result from the dance of the parents.

1

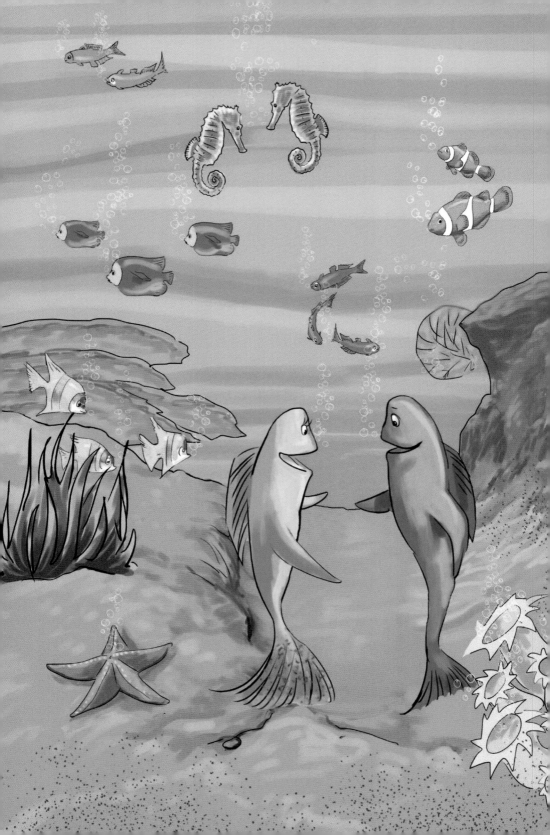

It happens like this:

When a dancing fish couple falls in love and decide to start their own family, they search out a whirlpool.

A whirlpool is a place in the ocean where the water goes round and round, neither too fast, nor too slow. A beautiful place where the fish like to play.

When they find the perfect spot, they start their beautiful dance.

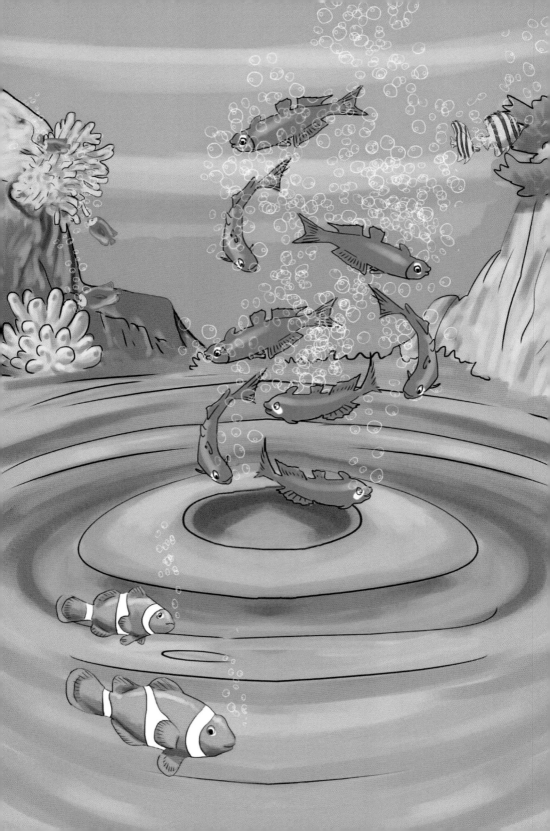

They dance and dance with each other until the lady Dancing Fish releases her eggs into the water, after which the gentleman releases his seed.

Gently, the whirlpool pulls the eggs and the seed along, causing it to make a dance of their own until somewhere during their dance an egg and a seed dance into each other - and a new Dancing Fish starts its amazing life journey.

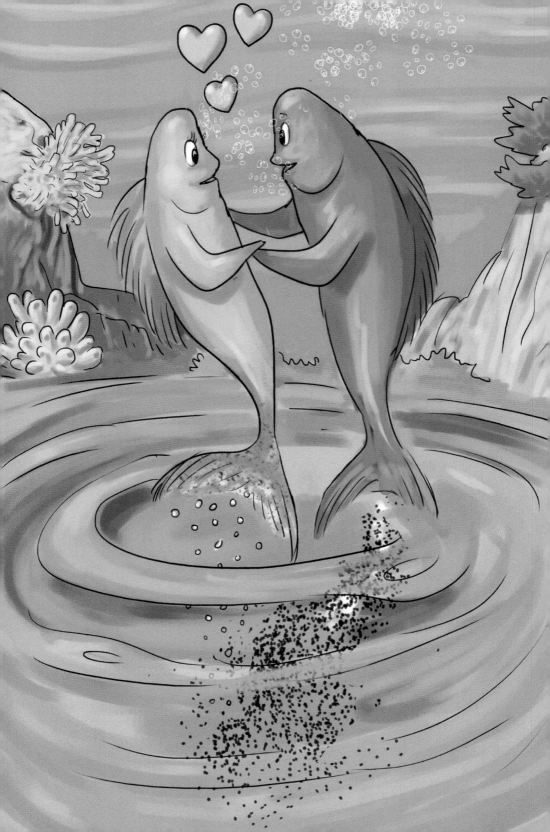

One day, a kind and clever crab was peacefully enjoying the beautiful ocean view, when he heard someone crying. The crying was so full of pain and sadness that he simply could not ignore it. He quietly moved closer to see who was crying so.

He saw a lady Dancing Fish, gently being held in the fins of her mate, who was desperately trying to console her, though he was crying too.

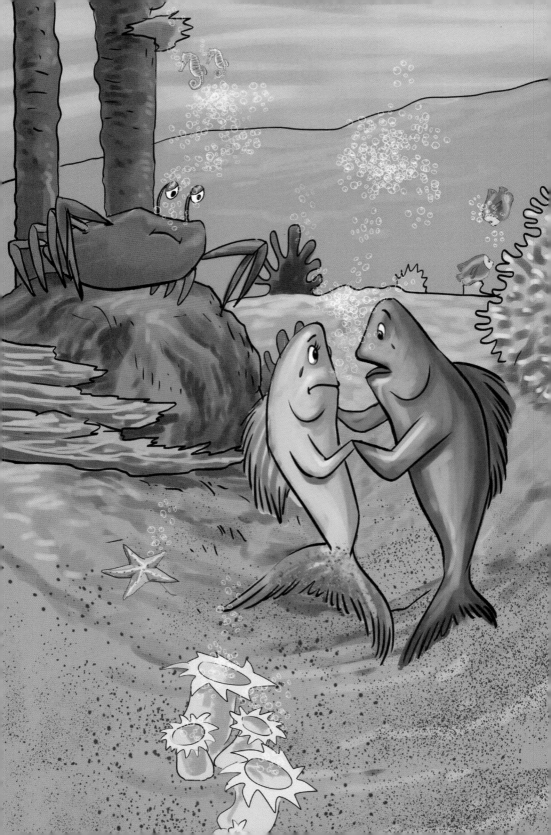

Normally the crab minded his own business, but this was too much for his kind heart to bear so he gently asked: "Why are you so sad dear Dancing Fish?"

"We cry because it seems we'll never have little Dancing Fish to love.

We've tried and tried, we don't know why we can't be parents too," the gentleman replied with a deep, sad, sigh.

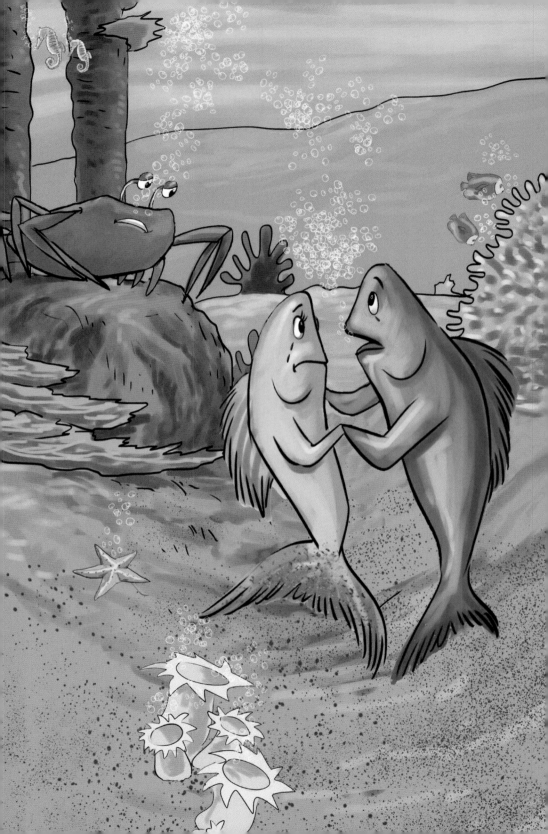

"Mmmm," said the crab, while scratching his head with one of his claws.

"Mmmm," he said again.

He was giving the matter serious thought. 'There must be a way,' he thought, 'there must be a way to replace their sadness with joy.'

After quite a while of thinking he said, "It could be your eggs, it could be your seed, it could be, mmmm..."

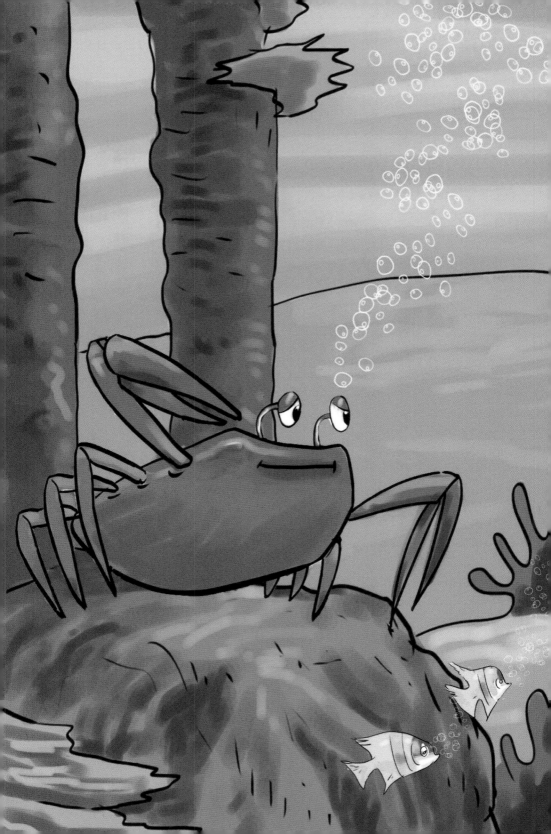

Then a very clever idea occurred to him

and he said excitedly:

"If you will ask for eggs and seed from

other Dancing Fish, I will gently take the

eggs in one claw, some seed in the other,

and swim to my quiet place behind the

big rock.

There I will make a little current go round

and round with my claws. The seed will

swirl and swirl around the eggs until an

egg and seed dance into each other, and

your new baby Dancing Fish is made!"

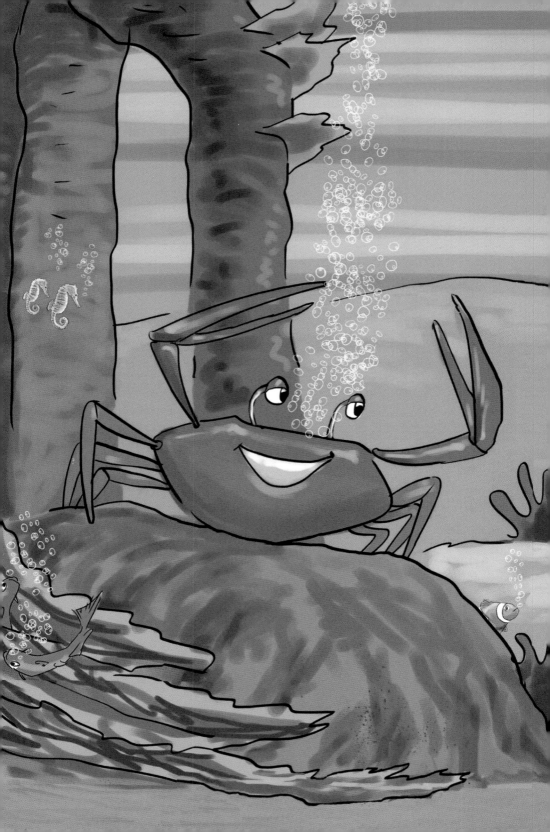

This idea was so strange, that the Dancing Fish forgot about crying, they just stared at the crab.

"Ask other Dancing Fish for eggs and seed?" the gentleman asked.

"Yes," the Clever Crab answered, "I'm sure you'll find Dancing Fish kind enough to do this for you."

"Making little Dancing Fish in such a unique way!" the lady whispered in wonder.

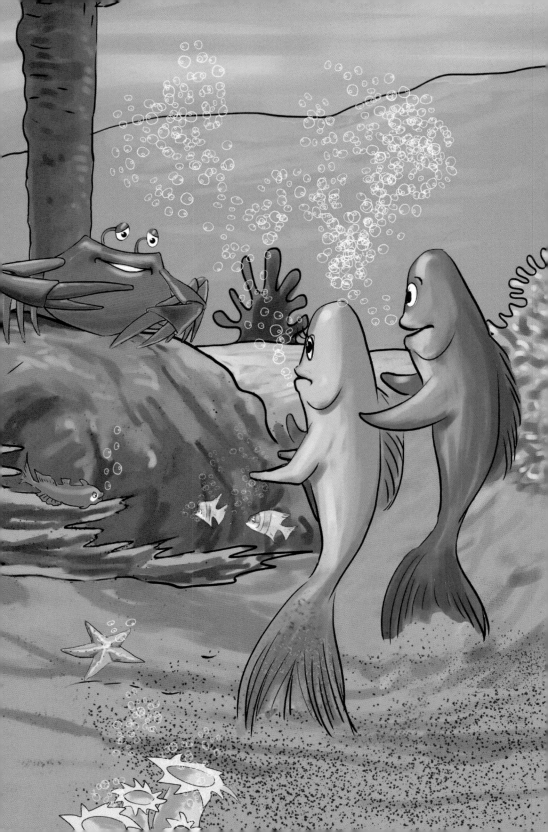

"But will it be our baby?" they asked.
"After all, you used the seed and eggs of
other Dancing Fish."

"My dear Dancing Fish" the crab said
patiently, "all creatures with personality
have two parts: the body and the person.

The body is the container for the person, a
'shell' if you will. That's all the body is, a
shell, nothing more, nothing less.
It's not important who makes the shell:
a shell is just a shell after all.

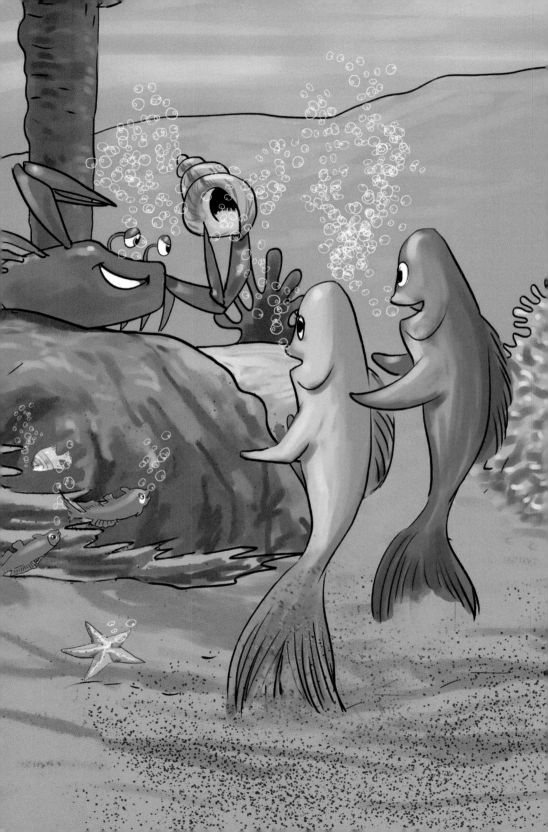

It may be pretty, or not so much.

It may be strong, or weak. It may be big,

or small. What does it matter?

It's just a shell.

It's the person living inside the shell who

is important, for it's the person who

makes the fish the kind of fish other sea

creatures want around, or not.

It's the person who makes the ocean a

better or worse place, a kinder, happier or

an unhappier place. It is the person who

counts, not the shell."

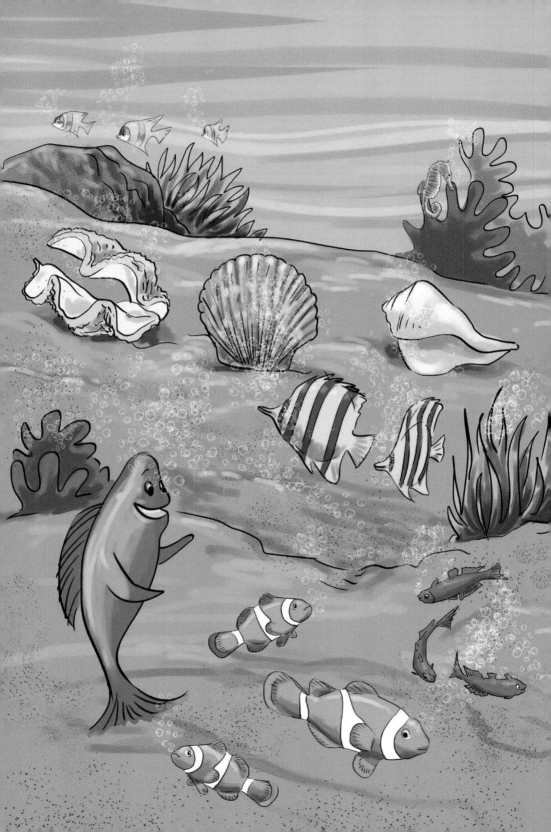

"It's the person living inside the shell who needs guidance, who needs training, who needs love, who needs to learn about life from wise and caring parents.

Will the two of you not be the best parents you could possibly be?" the Crab asked.

Both the Dancing Fish shook their heads up and down, saying:
"Yes, yes, we'll do our best."
"I knew it!" exclaimed the Crab happily.

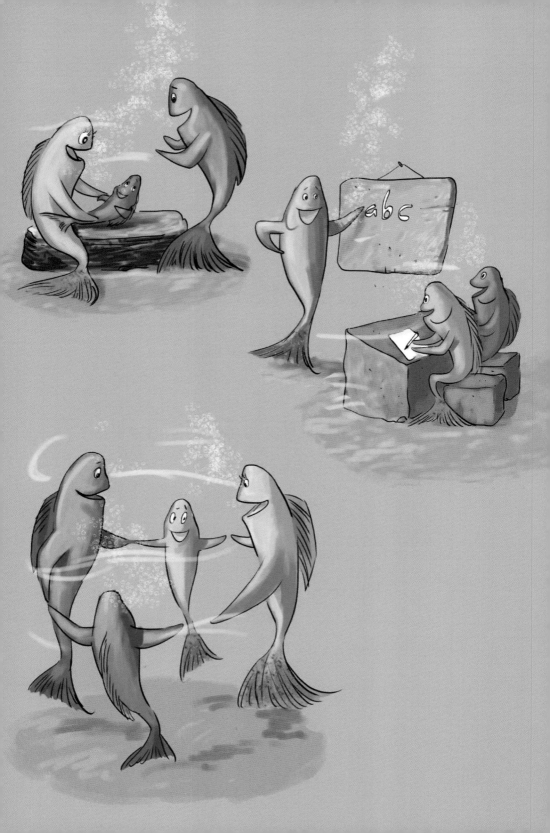

"Oh can this be true? Can this really be done?"

"It can be done, I know it can." The Clever Crab replied. He looked very confident. So confident in fact, that hope began to replace their sadness.

"Our own family," the lady Dancing Fish said happily.
"Our own family," the gentleman Dancing Fish echoed.
Their tears of sadness were replaced by smiles of joy.

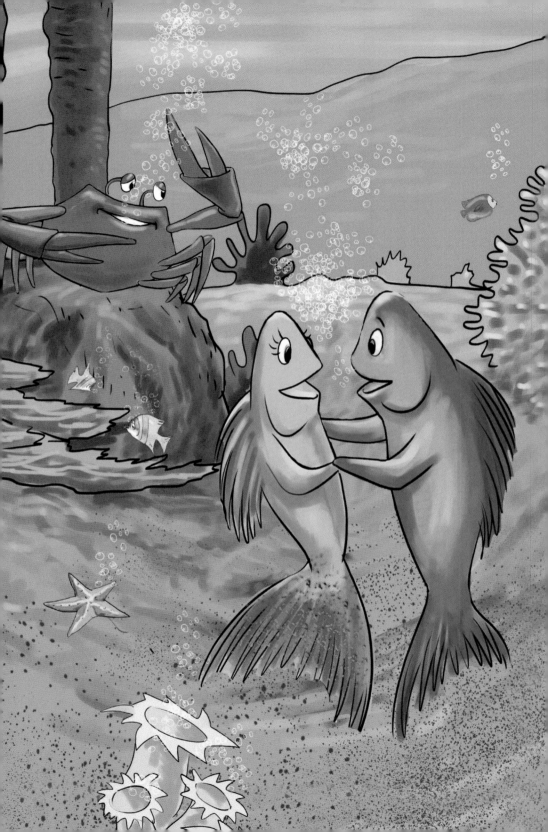

"And that's just what they did! Our parents asked other Dancing Fish for some of their eggs and seed.

The Clever Crab took the seed and eggs gently in his claws to his special place behind a rock. And just as he said he would, he made a little current go round and round till the eggs and seed danced together.

And so we were made in this very special way!" the little Dancing Fish explained.

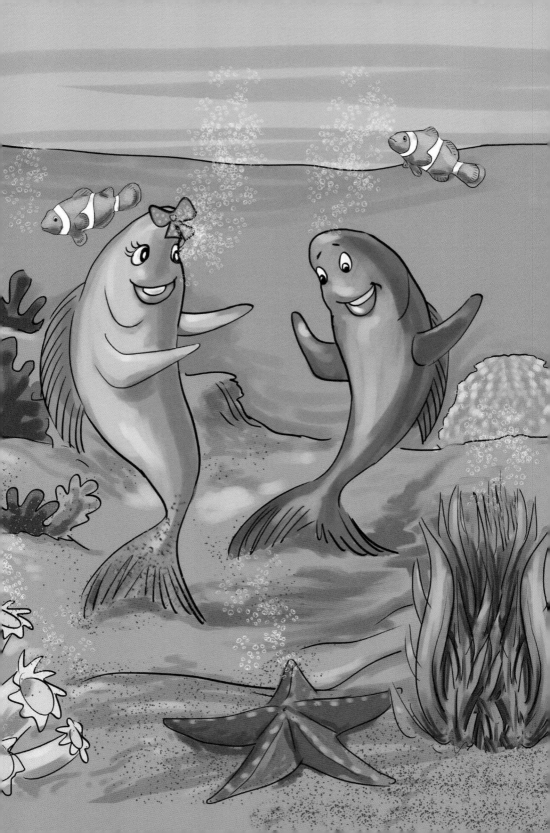

"With parents who wanted us so much and who love us so much, we've decided to become the kind of fish other sea creatures would be happy to have around."

The little Dancing Fish did indeed make others happy, but no one was as happy as their Mom and Dad!

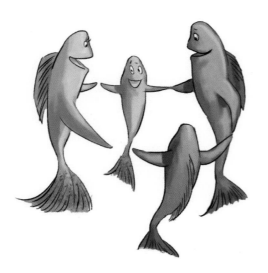

The End

Printed in Great Britain
by Amazon